The U-spot

By Michelle Tallia

PS-spot.com

ISBN-13: 978-1501045974
ISBN-10: 1501045970

This book comes with four additional bonus books. Your books are presented in this order:

Book #1

The PS-Spot Orgasm: Don't Wait Any Longer For This Kind of Pleasure

by Michelle Tallia

This book may make note of, or be linked to other websites which are not maintained by any party or parties involved with this book and/or its website (should it have one.) The writer and publisher of this book expressly disclaim all liability for the use or interpretation by others of information contained in this or hyperlinked Web sites listed in this book.

Anal stimulation runs the particular risk of spread of disease and all anal activity/penetration requires a high degree of sanitation, before, during and afterward. Make sure fingernails are well trimmed and hands are very clean before using them on/in a body.

There's an online videoclip showing how to find and stimulate the PS-Spot at www.orgasmarts.com/ps-spot **(Orgasm Arts). Please note, it shows naked female genitalia, so only look at it in private. The writer and publisher of this book are not associated with this graphic but very informative videoclip.**

Many women know what Perineal Massage is. Women often do this (or have it done to them) to lessen the physical trauma of pushing their babies out of their vagina. Perineal massage involves massaging the perineum (the area located between the anus and the vagina.) This practice is most often done during the final weeks of pregnancy. It protects against tears to the perineal during childbirth.

This book however is about a different perineal related activity.

Learning how to stimulate the female Perineal Sponge (or *PS-Spot* as it's often called) could provide an amazing treat for everybody involved. The PS-Spot can extend an orgasm, make orgasms happen quicker, make them more intense and/or create an orgasm on its own.

The PS-Spot is an often overlooked part of the female sexual anatomy and definitely worth investigating. If you're a man, knowing how to stimulate it (or even knowing of its existence) can really impress a woman. If you're a woman, as you have one, congratulations! Now let's put it to work.

Connected to the truly amazing clitoris is a network of nerves and blood vessels that branch into various clitoral structures. These include the spongy erectile bodies: *the Clitoral Bulbs, the Urethral Sponge and the*

Perineal Sponge. The woman's spongy erectile bodies aid intercourse by absorbing her blood like a sponge thus increasing their size and pushing on the vagina walls to make her vagina a tighter fit for the penis. (If one or more of a woman's spongy erectile bodies aren't working properly, it may be noticeable in intercourse as her vagina might not be as tight a fit as expected. This however is not thought to be a wide-spread problem.)

The Perineal Sponge (PS-Spot) is found in the lower genital area of women. Via a wealth of nerves, it's connected to the clitoris. It lies a little (½ to 1½ inches) beneath the perineum (the area between the vaginal and the anus.)

Internally the shaft of the clitoral system divides into two 'legs' that curve downward and look somewhat like a wishbone. These are called "crura", the Latin word for legs. You cannot see or feel these 'legs' but the perineal sponge is connected to the clitoral system largely by these. Mainly because of this connection the *Urethral Sponge* and the *Perineal Sponge* can provide sexual pleasure. (The urethral sponge (the U-spot) is discussed a bit more in depth later on and the author also has written a book on *U-spot sexual pleasure.*)

Both males and females have a *Perineal.* In males it's located where the penis starts (*which is located above the scrotum and called the "bulb of the penis"*) and the anus. In females, it's found between the vagina and anus, roughly 1.25 centimeters from the anus if you start your measurement from the vagina. (That figure can vary.)

As both sexes become sexually aroused, our bodies create substances that cause blood to rush to the genitals, where the blood expands specialized erectile tissue called "bulbs". Men have a single bulb (the bulb of the penis) and women have two bulbs beneath the inner lips of her vagina. If unaroused, normally you can't see or feel the bulbs, but as you're aroused they expand and the genitals become puffed out, creating the female clitoral erection and of course the male erection.

The perineal sponge is internal and often positioned an even distance between the vagina and anus. It's just beneath the perineum. As already noted the perineal sponge (the PS-spot) consists of female erectile tissue. When a woman is sexually stimulated, it fills with blood and becomes enlarged just as a man's penis and a woman's clitoris does during arousal. As it becomes swollen with blood, it compressing the outer third of the vagina creating a tighter fit and thus additional stimulation for the penis. (The *Urethral Sponge* does the same but at a different location of the vagina.)

The PS-spot can also be stimulated through the anus. If you're a fan of anal sex then it's suggested you make a particular effort to stimulate PS-spot during anal sex. Some or more women who orgasm during anal sex may be doing so largely from having their perineal sponge stimulated.

These orgasms may be accompanied with ejaculation and may feel similar to orgasms from G-spot stimulation.

A description of the PS-spot comes from sexuality educator Ashley Manta. "If you take your tongue and feel the skin on the roof of your mouth, right behind your {front} teeth, that's what the {stimulated} perineal sponge feels like. It's a little firm, with ridges."

One way to look at it is that if a women is sitting, she has the G-spot on the roof (top) of her vaginal canal and the PS-spot on the floor (bottom) of her vaginal canal.

Note that the PS-Spot is not the same as the "P-Spot" as the P-spot is short for "Prostate Spot" and thus obviously associated only with men, (where the PS-Spot is associated only with women.)

It has been reported that some Tantric sex followers refer to the PS-Spot as the "Cali spot".

How to Stimulate the Perineal Sponge and Have a PS-Spot Orgasm

The PS-spot is innately erogenous tissue with a large number of nerve endings. It can be stimulated via the vagina or via the rectum (anus), or by stimulating it using both orifices at the same time.

A number of methods can be incorporated to achieve (or at least attempt to achieve) your PS-spot orgasm. You can use fingers (make sure to trim those finger nails down), a variety of toys, particularly curved end vibrating toys, non-vibrating curved end toys, a penis, or a combination. The PS-spot may also be sensitive to massage/pressure when applied directly to the outer perineum (the skin between the vagina and anus.)

Most often however the woman has to first be sexually excited to get the desired impact from PS-spot stimulation. In other words first get aroused then start the PS-spot stimulation.

PS-spot stimulation can be accomplished by masturbation or by a lover.

There's an online videoclip showing how to find and stimulate the PS-Spot at www.orgasmarts.com/ps-spot **(Orgasm Arts). Please note, it shows naked female genitalia, so only look at it in private. The writer and publisher of this book are not associated with this graphic but very informative videoclip.**

Often it's best to simultaneously stimulate the PS-spot from both top and bottom by using well manicured, very clean fingers and/or toys in both her anus and vagina at the same time.

For simplicity, let's start with accessing the PS-spot by only using one of those entrances at a time.

1) Often, *(a)* well manicured, very clean fingers, or *(b)* very clean curved-tip toys, are best for attaining sexual pleasure from the perineal sponge, (the PS-spot). This is compared to intercourse, though many women get PS-spot orgasms from intercourse.

2) Many of the same suggestions for stimulating the G-spot holds true for stimulating the PS-spot, except the PS-Spot typically is not as far into the vagina.

To look for the G-spot, after she's sexually aroused, insert one or two fingers in the vagina with your palm facing her vagina. Gently bend your fingers up towards her head so that they stroke the front wall (thus the upper wall if she's lying on her back) of her vagina. You may feel a raised spot or series of ridges, or nothing in particular. The woman may find this extremely pleasurable, or may have an urge to urinate, or both. Stroking this area with varying degrees of pressure will most likely tell the woman if she's got a G-spot or not.

To find the PS-spot using this type of method, remember that it's on the opposite part of her vagina so the hand doing the stimulating/searching likely will need to turn 180 degrees. Also it is only ½ to 1½ inches in to the vagina versus 2-3 inches in to the vagina as are most G-spots.

The G-Spot, or Grafenberg Spot is named after its discoverer, a German gynecologist called Ernst Grafenberg. It's defined as a bean-shaped area of the vagina that when stimulated, can lead to strong sexual arousal, powerful orgasms and female ejaculation. It's sometimes referred to as the *Goddess Spot*. 1940s research into the female orgasm led to the discovery that the female's urethral tube, which lies on top of the vagina, is surrounded by erectile tissue similar to that found in the male penis. When the female becomes sexually aroused, this tissue swells. In the G-spot zone this expansion results in a small protrusion through the vaginal wall that protrudes into the vaginal canal. It's this raised patch that is, according to Grafenberg, "a primary erotic zone, perhaps more important than the clitoris." {That is something that has been proven to be incorrect.} He stated that its significance was lost when the 'missionary position' became a dominant feature of human sexual behavior as there are other sexual positions that are more efficient at stimulating this erogenous zone (the G-spot.)

The term "G-spot" was not used by Grafenberg himself, he called it "an erotic zone", which actually is a better description of it. Unfortunately, the modern use of "G-spot" as a popular term has led to some misunderstandings. Some women mistakenly believe that there is a 'magic sexual pleasure button' that can be activated at any time to get great pleasure. The truth is that the G-spot is a sexually sensitive patch in the vaginal wall that protrudes slightly only when the glands surrounding the urethral tube have become swollen (mainly the *urethral sponge*). Importantly, the woman needs to be significantly sexually stimulated first to get it to do that.

For a while the sexual establishment denied the existence of such a thing. Sexual politics had reared its ugly head. (Remember this was in the 1940s and 50s. Women back then still weren't expected to get great pleasure from sex and many questioned whether a vaginal orgasm was even possible. They tended to believe a clitoral orgasm was possible though.)

There have been reports of women undergoing 'G-spot enhancement'. This involves injecting collagen into the G-spot zone to enlarge it (thus pushing it further into the vagina so it interacts with the thrusting penis more.) According to one source, "One of the latest procedures to catch on is *G-spot injection*. The idea is that this will increase its sensitivity and give you better orgasms."

The fact is that a large number of women are getting enhanced sexual pleasure and/or orgasms by stimulating the area where the G-spot is suppose to be but there remains a major controversy as to whether the G-spot even exists. The writer of this book assumes the G-spot exists but has no conclusive proof.

Locating and/or Stimulating Your PS-Spot via the Vagina

If a woman is lying on her back, the *back (posterior)* wall of the vagina is the part of her vagina that is closest to the bed, and the *lower* part of her vagina is the part of her vagina that's closest to the vagina's entrance.

As the PS-spot is erectile tissue, typically the woman needs to be turned on sexually for it to be most significantly activated (filled with blood and thus 'erect'.) By activated I mean getting firmer to the touch. This can be accomplished in the usual manner, through breast stimulation, clitoral stimulation or even kissing depending on how quickly and easily she gets sexually stimulated. In other words in many cases it doesn't work as well to start playing with her PS-spot if she isn't already turned on.

When only using the vagina for PS-spot stimulation, (versus using both the vagina and anus simultaneously,) the PS-spot can be accessed via the *lower back* wall of the vagina. It's between ½ to 1½ inches into the vagina. Your *well manicured, very clean* finger or toy enters the vagina and pushes down toward the anus. Start by pushing down only a half inch in, then a little further in until she feels the stimulation. (Typically it's not more than 1½ inches into the vagina.) You flick/move your finger in a manner that gives her the most pleasure. If you're using a toy perhaps sliding it back and forth a bit will do the trick, particularly if it's a vibrating toy. However please note, many women simply don't have a PS-spot, or at least one at that time of her life.

If a woman wants to try to stimulate her perineal sponge during intercourse, either with a penis or dildo, she should position herself in a manner that directs the phallic implement of choice toward the back (thus bottom if she's laying on her back,) wall of the vagina. Three recommended sexual positions are:

*The missionary position
*The woman-on-top position
*Seated and facing each other.

You want to do the opposite of what works best for targeting the G-spot. For instance doggy style vaginal intercourse is a good G-spot sex position but not as good for the PS-spot.

Locating and/or Stimulating Your PS-Spot via the Anus

The rectum lies against the sacrum (lower backbone) in a gentle curve down to the anal opening which as you know is penetrated during anal sex. The front (anterior) wall of the rectum and rear wall of the vagina, and the thin layer of tissue between them, are together called the *rectovaginal septum* (or wall).

Anally the perineal sponge can be accessed via the front wall of the rectum. (If a woman is lying on her back, the *front wall* of the rectum is that which is closest to her vagina.)

Use a *well manicured, very clean finger* (and remember to keep anything that has touched her anus, away from her vagina. That's important!)

There's an online videoclip showing how to find and stimulate the PS-Spot at www.orgasmarts.com/ps-spot **(Orgasm Arts). Please note, it shows naked female genitalia, so only look at it in private. The writer and publisher of this book are not associated with this graphic but very informative videoclip.**

As the man's prostate is stimulated from being taken anally (as that's his *P-spot*), conversely a woman's PS-spot can be stimulated from being taken anally.

A reason the G-spot feels good when touched is because it stimulates the clitoris from the clitoris' underside. The clitoris isn't just what you see on the outside. It actually goes roughly a couple inches inside of a woman.

The PS-spot is located closer to the rectum than the G-spot, though further from the clitoris. (but remember the PS-spot is connected to the powerful clitoral system via the clitoris' crura.)

1) When testing to see if a woman has a PS-spot, it could be best to first explore for, and/or stimulate the potential PS-spot location with a thinner sex toy, or normal size finger. (Trim the finger nail!!!) Remember its located ½ to 1½ inches in from the vagina's entrance. A wider sex toy, or a penis, should the receiver not be used to it, could cause physical anxiety and/or trauma that takes away from the PS-spot sexual enhancement experience.

2) Generally speaking, fingers or curved-tip toys are best for applying pressure on the perineal sponge, whether insertion is occurring via the vagina or via the anus. In many cases though, simple insertion by a penis *into the anus* versus the vagina can have more success stimulating the PS-spot than simple insertion by a penis into the vagina. Chances are good that

if a woman orgasms from anal sex alone, at least part of that is from PS-spot stimulation.

3) Don't forget about finger vibrators. These little vibrators slide onto your finger and well, I think you can imagine how well these can work.

As previously noted the PS-spot is located between the rectum and vagina so when insertion of a toy or phallus is occurring in the anus, the emphasis/pressure should be on the part the rectum closest to the vagina.

Locating and/or Stimulating Your PS-Spot by Utilizing the Anus and Vagina at the Same Time.

This is the preferred way to search for and activate her PS-spot, but remember anything that touches the anus cannot touch the vagina!

1) The woman should be sexually excited so the erectile tissue, which includes the perineal sponge, has filled or is filling with blood. This makes the PS-spot easier to find and more sensitive.
2) Use plenty of lubricant.
3) Use a *well manicured, very clean finger/thumb to* enter her vagina and another finger/thumb to enter her anus at the same time.
4) Massage, rub and/or vibrate the PS-spot (which is between the two openings) simultaneously from insertion into both the top and bottom 'holes'. The PS-spot is located only ½ to 1½ inches in from their entrances.
5) Just because she didn't orgasm from it this time or not get a great deal of pleasure doesn't mean she won't when you do it again in the future.

While having intercourse, one of the parties can stimulate the PS-spot through the unoccupied opening, or even the outside of the *Perineal* (which is the skin between the vagina and anus.)

The Perineal Sponge may respond to pressure from the outside of the perineal body.

The perineal sponge may respond to pressure from outside the body too, though this could depend on how much fat and muscle is in between it and your skin. Try a vibrator that you would normally use on your clitoris and press and move it against the skin that is located equidistant between the vagina and anus. Chances are good pushing up will help. With experimentation you can determine the best way to stimulate the PS-spot this way, if your PS-spot can even can be stimulated this way.

Stimulating the Urethral Sponge

The perineal sponge is not the same as the urethral sponge. Like the perineal sponge the urethral sponge is a spongy cushion of erectile tissue found in the lower genital area of women. It sits against both the pubic bone and vaginal wall and surrounds the urethra. Its job however is much the same as the perineal sponge. With sexual stimulation, it engorges itself with blood and makes a tighter more pleasurable fit for the penis. It is however closer to the clitoris.

The G-spot is located in the urethral sponge and one theory is that as the urethral sponge engorges itself with blood from sexual excitement, it pushes down on the G-spot area which more fully activates the G-spot's clitoral nerve connection, giving the woman sexual pleasure.

The urethral sponge provides women with the "U-spot". The U-spot can be located in different parts of the urethral sponge; its size can vary from woman to woman. (Unfortunately many women don't have a pleasurable U-spot to start out with.) The U-spot isn't the same as the G-spot but the G-spot can be located in the often bigger U-Spot.

The urethral sponge encompasses sensitive nerve endings connected to the clitoris. It can be stimulated through the front wall of the vagina. Some women experience intense pleasure from stimulation of the urethral sponge (U-spot) while others find the sensation irritating. The urethral sponge surrounds clitoral nerves, and since the two are so closely interconnected, stimulation of the clitoris may stimulate the nerve endings of the urethral sponge and vice versa. Some women get U-spot pleasure from the rear-entry position of *vaginal intercourse* (whether she's laying on her stomach or on her hands and knees) as the penis is often angled slightly downward and can stimulate the front wall of the vagina, and in turn the urethral sponge.

If you have a pleasurable U-spot you want to get to know it better as there is documented evidence of women getting earth-shattering orgasms from it as women have with the PS-spot.

Conclusion

Women, enhance your sexual pleasure with a part of your body you already have and likely are not even using!

Is the PS-Spot also one of your hot spots? I certainly hope so and for many people it is. (Incidentally if the G-spot isn't a hotspot for you, don't assume the PS-Spot won't be also, as actually often it is.) Unfortunately there's no guarantee that optimal utilization of any sexual part of your body will make you scream like a ban chi. The important thing is that you explored an erroneous zone in your body (and there are others) to make sure you can be all you can be.

There's an online videoclip showing how to find and stimulate the PS-Spot at <u>www.orgasmarts.com/ps-spot</u> (Orgasm Arts). Please note, it shows naked female genitalia, so only look at it in private. The writer and publisher of this book are not associated with this graphic but very informative videoclip.

Guys, an easy, cheap way to delay ejaculation is: anti-hemorrhoidal and anesthetic ointments. I know a man who used NUPERCAINAL for that purpose. It's an over-the-counter medicine and readily available at many drug stores. I suggest however that you only put *very little* on as it's very potent. You want to mainly put it on the underside of the tip of the penis. It will be absorbed by the skin after a while. *Guys you'll have to test it yourself to see what the best amount for your use is because if you put too much on (which is easy to do) you might not feel her stroking you in an attempt to make you hard.* Please note this disclaimer. I do not know if there are any side effects to its use and though I don't know of anybody having a problem with it, it's possible. Contact a physician before using it.

The End

Book #2
The A-spot Orgasm: The Elusive Super Orgasm

By Michelle Tallia

Copyright © 2014

PS-spot.com

Anal stimulation runs the particular risk of spread of disease and all anal activity/penetration requires a high degree of sanitation, before, during and afterward. Make sure fingernails are well trimmed and hands are very clean before using them on/in a body.

The A-spot Orgasm: The Elusive Super Orgasm

Anal stimulation runs the particular risk of spread of disease and all anal activity/penetration requires a high degree of sanitation, before, during and afterward. Make sure fingernails are well trimmed and hands are very clean before using them on/in a body.

The A-Spot is located high up in the innermost point of the vagina, (the anterior or front wall if she's facing you.) It's in front of, and above the cervix. If you continue on the anterior surface beyond the G-spot you'll round the bend to the back side of the pubic bone and the cervix. The cervix is the innermost spot of the vagina and should be handled very delicately. The cervix is the narrow part that protrudes slightly into the vagina, leaving a circular recess around itself. The front part of this recess is called the anterior fornix, and where you want to go. Pressure on it often produces rapid lubrication of the vagina, even in women who are not normally sexually responsive. To probe this zone an *A-spot (AFE) vibrator* should be long, thin and curved upward towards its end. Ideally it should be longer than your typical curved tip G-spot vibrator.

The A-spot is also referred to as the *Epicentre, AFE-zone, Anterior Fornix Erogenous Zone, Cul-de-Sac* and *Vaginal Fornix*. This is a patch of sensitive tissue at the inner end of the vaginal tube between the cervix and the bladder. It's often described as the 'female degenerated prostate'. (Thus it's the female equivalent of the male prostate, just as the clitoris is the female equivalent of the male penis.) Direct stimulation of this spot can produce:

- Violent orgasmic contractions
- The sensation of needing to pee
- Female ejaculation
- Irritation
- Do nothing at all.

For those that like it (and there are many who do) it can be practically life-changing. As another plus, unlike clitoral orgasms, the A-spot often doesn't suffer from post-orgasmic over-sensitivity.

The A-Spot was discovered by DR. CHUA CHEE ANN of Malaysia in the 90s. (www.aspot-pioneer.com). The good doctor discovered it while looking for a way to treat vaginal dryness. Stimulating this spot typically causes high arousal and natural lubrication in women, which as previously noted can include female ejaculation.

The A-spot is located on the same wall of the vagina as is the G-Spot (the anterior or front wall if she is facing you.) Remember that the vagina is on average about 3-4 inches long but with sexual stimulation it can get quite a bit longer. It's often difficult for a woman to find and/or stimulate her own A-spot due to its recessed location. That may be solved with the use of an A-spot (AFE) vibrator or a long, preferably thin, curved-tip dildo.

The fornix is the area right around the cervix; assuming you still have one. The anterior fornix would be the area in front of the cervix. If, for surgical reasons, you no longer have a fornix, you probably no longer have the A-spot either.

Some people theorize that the A-spot is one of the things that give some women strong orgasms during anal sex.

The A-spot may also be why some women have powerful orgasms if her partner just goes deep with his penis and stays there jiggling. If condoms are not being used (something the author is not suggesting), then that may be a reason that some women orgasm so hard when the ejaculate lands deep inside her, i.e. on her A-spot. (Chances are good also that it's from the general sexual stimulation.)

Note that during stimulation she could feel the need to urinate, whether she actually needs to or not (and more often than not she won't need to.) This feeling can go away at anytime and then, assuming she's stimulated correctly, mainly she'll feel sexual pleasure. Another possibility is that she'll find it uncomfortable. Maybe it's because her lover is not gentle enough or maybe it's just not her thing.

Best sexual intercourse positions are the *woman on top position* and *the missionary position* with her legs pinned to her chest, or pinned deep along her sides. Make sure he's all the way inside of her then he should try moving the tip of his penis as much as possible. Perhaps he's long enough to slide over the pubic bone, jiggle the top of his penis and essentially slide over the A-spot, stimulating it. Unfortunately the A-spot is not located straight up into the vagina but instead is a little inside the curve of the cervix. However the skin in the inner part of the vagina that the penis moves against could connect to the A-spot indirectly, providing sexual stimulation. Unfortunately it's doubtful that he'll be able to touch the A-spot with his penis because as previously noted it's located just passed the curve of the cervix.

A-spot stimulation experts note that it may be necessary to stimulate the A-spot for at least a few minutes a day to build up to more intense use. If a woman achieves a powerful A-spot orgasm, she could find that her strongest orgasms of her life come from it. A lover that's proficient in how to stimulate the A-spot will almost certainly provide a memorable sexual experience for a woman. Do note however that it can take time and multiple attempts for a woman to achieve optimal results, and sadly some women never do. Be patient! Those women that have a patient, delicate and knowledgeable A-spot trainer statistically usually get pleasure from it.

More tips on what to do:

1) First getting her sexually stimulated is a good idea. This can be from foreplay and/or actual intercourse but remember with sexual stimulation typically one gets increased length of the vagina (which pushes where we have to go further away.) Some women find this 'pre' stimulation more helpful in getting A-spot orgasms than others.

2) Make sure she's relaxed and comfortable. Have her lay on her back with her knees back as far as they can go, (against her chest or each leg off to her sides.) Tie her legs back if such a thing is allowed in your relationship. While in these positions, as the A-spot is located just past the back end of the vagina, the A-spot is effectively brought forward some.

3) With palm up (the bigger the hand, often the better), slide your longest very well manicured, clean and lubricated finger deep into her vagina to her cervix, (the entrance to her womb). It may feel like a little dog's nose. It might instead feel more rubbery than just fleshy and like there are elastic bands under the surface. Perhaps now you should add another finger.

Once you've arrived at a spot to test, you should try a 'come-hither' motion against that spot with your inserted finger (as if you were using your finger to signal someone to come towards you). You may need to try still more spots.

Be ready for her orgasm as she can buck while in the throngs of passion. You'll likely need to hold her down as she moves about and her hips thrust about. An implement in her anus holding her down and/or a finger or two from your other hand pushing down on the posterior (back) side of the vagina (if she is laying on her back,) could help do that. Tying her pelvis securely down bondage style can be a very good idea.

Once her lover knows the location of her A-spot (something that could take more than one try,) sliding in and manipulating a vibrator (versus using fingers) likely is the easier thing to do.

4) As it is often easier for a lover to give a woman an A-spot orgasm than for her to do it herself, she may want it quite a bit, but it is work for her lover and the person giving it gets little if any sexual pleasure. Maybe her lover can give it as a treat and/or a reward.

Barbara Keesling from Cal State Fullerton wrote the important book related to this *Super Sexual Orgasm: Discover the Ultimate Pleasure Spot*

The Cul-de-Sac. She noted, "It's called light-socket sex... Seriously, you get the fireworks sensation of the lights behind your eyes. You get unusual sensations in your retina that we would call, like, fireworks. You get shooting colors. And it also makes you weak in the knees when you go to stand up afterward. And it also gives you a kind of uhhh, uhhh panting type of sensation."

Best of times to all!

The End

Book #3

The Absolutely Essential Guide to Erotic Breast Massage

Michelle Tallia

Copyright (C) 2014

The specialized breast massage discussed in this book can give a woman a surprising amount of pleasure. If her lover is unavailable to pleasure her this way women can easily give themselves *Extreme Pleasure Breast Massage*, and it's something women can do to themselves for the rest of their lives.

There are a many positions a woman's body can be in to receive this specialized and very sexually arousing breast massage. For this example though, let's have her sitting up and at least topless. Do note however that as she gets more and more aroused, she'd probably prefer to be naked so one or both of you can access her pubic area with fingers or toys while she's experiencing Extreme Pleasure Breast Massage.

For this position the massager sits behind her with his/her chest up against her back. If it's okay with who is getting the massage, I suggest the massager be naked as many women will lose control at some point when getting Extreme Pleasure Breast Massage and be anxiously reaching behind their lower backs to play with the massager's privates. If a woman has never experienced this type of erotic massage before, she in particular may react with callous abandon.

Before placing yourselves in any of the massage positions, you'll need to have readily available a good supply of quality lotion, massage oil or hair conditioner (yes the stuff you might put on your hair. Thicker hair conditioner is often better and the cheaper brands might work just as well.)

If using lotion, try to use some brand of non-desensitizing lotion. (Most lotion's ingredients include desensitizers to dull the pain of dry skin and other irritations. These desensitizers can at least partially desensitize breasts, thus cutting down on the breast's capacity to provide pleasure.) Baby lotions at dollar stores may be good ones to try but lotions tend to vary by brand. Optimally you want the massaging medium to stay slippery as long as possible and, not cause any irritation of course. Cold lotion/oil/conditioner on breasts can provide an unwelcome jolt so if warming is necessary, warm the lotion/oil/conditioner up ahead of time using the microwave oven, or by setting it in hot water. Make sure the top is loosened somewhat incase it warms up too much and creates steam. (You can also rub together blobs of it in your hands to warm it up.) Always have an ample amount of this massage oil/lotion/hair conditioner nearby as well as small towels to wipe it off of your hands and her breasts after the massage is over. It would be best to wash it off.

Put a sizeable glob of massage oil/lotion/conditioner on each of your hands, rubbing it all over the palms of your hands to spread it out, as well as warm it if it's not yet warm. Then put your well lubricated hands on her breasts, *but not yet on her nipples and areolas*. This is because those provide the most pleasure and thus the best is saved for last!

It is so important that the massager make sure to keep his/her massaging hands *very* well lubricated. When the oil or lotion is breaking down the massager will feel stickiness developing. **It is now time to put more massage oil/lotion/conditioner on!** The rule of thumb is that you can't lubricate your hands and her breasts too much!

Also the massager needs to make sure his/her nails and skin of their hands are smooth. Trim and file your fingernails and that kind of thing, to as short and smooth as possible. Otherwise she (the person receiving the massage) might feel them as they rub against her sensitive skin. She can even get hurt by them because as she is in the thongs of ecstasy, she might not realize that they are hurting her, so make sure to watch out for her and take care of this situation.

Typically the massage will provide three levels of pleasure. Massaging the fleshy part of her breast (but not massaging her areolas and nipples) should give her pronounced and very welcome pleasure; of course the faster her breasts are massaged the more pleasure she'll get.

Including her areolas in the massaging will increase her pleasure a lot. But massaging her nipples will really get her going.

Below (and not in order of importance) are suggestions to optimize the breast massage.

* Start from the bottom of her breasts (where the breasts meet her torso) and work your way slowly higher up to just below her areolas. You can move your hands at varying speeds but typically the faster you massage the more pleasure she'll get.

* Simultaneously circle her boobs with each hand. Start out by using limited pressure on the breasts while utilizing only one finger, then gradually work your way up to utilizing all your fingers. Go clockwise then counterclockwise (or vice-versa.) Remember, *leave her nipples and areolas alone as much as possible until she's practically (or literally) begging for you to massage them.* Sure you will "bump" into them from time to time as you massage around them. Those bumps will give her a delicious taste of what's to come.

* At its base, wrap each hand around a single breast then run your well lubricated hands around and along that breast in a steady spiraling motion up the breasts in the direction of her nipples, until you reach the edge of her areolas. Of course you can go in the opposite direction also (starting from just below her areolas and working your way down to where her boobs meets her torso.)

* Place one hand on the base of one breast; the back of the hand should be facing her head. Put your other hand on the base of her *other* breast, the back of it should be facing her legs. Slide your well lubricated hands from left to right and then vice-versa, across and along both breasts.

* At its base, take each breast in a well lubricated hand and with increasing speed pull up from the base of her breast toward the nipple until your fingers reach the edge of the areolas (or if you're already playing with her areolas and/or nipples, go all the way to her nipples.) Then do the opposite and slide your hands back down from the top of her breasts to the breast's base (where you started from.) Repeat this procedure many, many times.

* Tease her by sliding only your well lubricated, manicured fingertips over her breasts, wiggling your fingers.

* Instead of the above, perhaps for a minute or more, you'd like to start the festivities by teasing her breasts by only briefly touching them here and there using only the tips of your fingers.

* Concentrate your efforts on only one well lubricated breast; wrap both hands around it, kneading it, pulling it and twisting it.

As previously discussed, it's strongly suggested that you take your time before playing with her areolas and then nipples. This is because she will still get a good deal of pleasure from having the 'areola and nipple-less' massage. I for one require that she even beg you to play with her nipples--because as we know this is where the breasts offer the most pleasure.

Before finally massaging her nipples (admittedly you will "bump" into them periodically,) I would suggest waiting until she is already well stimulated. You may stroke her anticipation by whispering in her ear that you're about to play with her nipples, then suddenly do it! She may scream with delight as an orgasm overcomes her.

Playing with her nipples is typically the high point of the massage. She'll likely be getting the most pleasure now. (Again, the faster your well-lubricated fingers move around her nipples, the more pleasure she's likely to get.)

Okay massagers you now have a choice, you can immediately start massaging her nipples fast and hard, driving her crazy, or start massaging them slowly, then progressively massaging them faster and faster until she screams in ecstasy. If you're going to massage them fast immediately, as is the first option, many women will start their orgasm then (if they haven't already.)

Don't forget you can let her use a vibrator on herself as you massage her and thus it's suggested you keep a vibrator within her arm's reach. Believe me she'll find it if it's there.

Because so often the woman you're massaging will get so aroused from all this, that with both hands she'll instinctively reach around her lower back to play with the massager's pubic area. She then will not have a free hand to use the vibrator on herself. (Of course both your hands are busy giving her Extreme Pleasure Breast Massage.) A way to counter this is to secure a vibrator with white medical tape (the type used to hold gauge and cotton to cuts etc.) over her most sexually sensitive pubic area. (Perhaps it would be helpful if she keeps her panties on for extra support.) If you do this, more women will orgasm while you are giving her Extreme Pleasure Breast Massage.

Remember guys her nipples can get tender after orgasm and need to be left alone for at least a bit of time.

As is obvious, ladies, you can give yourself Extreme Pleasure Breast Massage in the privacy of your own bedroom.

After the massage, ladies your breasts tend to become firmer for a while and often they'll feel quite good for hours.

The following is another way of giving this massage, (told from the perspective of the kinky dominant massager.)

I will tell you to stand up and we will go to the bed (if we're not already there.) I will set the bed up so I am sitting with my back against the headboard of the bed and you are laying in front of me face-down on cushions (on the bed) with your head positioned so you can easily suck on my penis and play with my scrotum.

Also I'll put a roughly 3' x 3' sheet of plastic under your upper body to keep the massage lotion/oil/hair conditioner from going on the bed covers.

Perhaps I will also tie your hands together and perhaps then also to the headboard. If I do that though I will make sure there is enough slack in the rope for your hands to still move freely around my penis and scrotum while you suck. If your hands are tied to the headboard, I will be sitting on the rope as my butt will be in-between your bound hands and the headboard which your hands are tied to.

Your breasts will now be positioned, thanks to these cushions, just above the ground. As you suck on my penis, I will generously lubricate (and keep lubricated,) your breasts with some brand of preferably non-desensitizing massaging medium. I will warm the lotion/oil/hair conditioner up ahead of time or rub it in my hands to warm it up, if warming is necessary. I will then massage your breasts. (Many lotions put desensitizers in them to dull the pain of dry skin. These can at least partially desensitize breasts thus cutting down on the breast's capacity to provide pleasure.) I will continue for a long time to massage your lubricated breasts as you suck on my penis. (Remember to always keep the massager's hands well lubricated! The two of you will quickly notice that the nipples respond with the most pleasure from this massage.)

Using a yardstick type implement, I can reach across your back and spank you as you suck. Obviously one should make sure the woman can handle being spanked while sucking. Most can, depending on the intensity of the spanking and how hard she's already orgasming.

The End

The U-spot

By Michelle Tallia

Copyright © 2014

Book #4

PS-spot.com

ISBN-13: 978-1501045974
ISBN-10: 1501045970

The U-spot is one of the pressure points on the female urethral sponge. The "U" is short for urethral, or urethra. Not all women have a U-spot (or U-spots) that can give them pleasure and many will need numerous attempts to find it and/or get optimal pleasure from its stimulation.

(Note, while some websites will also call the U-spot the "Cul-de-sac", that is not a correct synonym for it. The "Cul-de-sac" is a synonym for the A-spot, a particularly powerful erogenous zone located just inside the vaginal entrance to the cervix. See the book *"The A-spot Orgasm: The Elusive Super Orgasm"*, also by Michelle Tallia.)

Let's start by getting some background information.

Erectile tissue

Erectile tissue is body tissue containing numerous tiny spaces (erectile capillaries) that can fill up with blood. This hardening makes the organ more sensitive and harder. Erectile tissue is best known for being in the ear, vestibular bulbs, penis, perineal sponge, urethral sponge, and nose.

Parts of the body can enlarge without the use of erectile tissue. These 'parts' include the nipples, vagina, labia minora (inner lips) and the urethra. (Nipple erection comes from the contraction of smooth muscle. It's the same reflex that causes goose bumps.)

Women have a network of connected erectile tissue organs. These primarily are the vestibular bulbs, the clitoris, the urethral sponge and the perineal sponge. Female arousal and/or orgasm might occur by stimulating any of these connected organs (or in other ways of course.) One reason pleasure is obtained from non-clitoral erectile tissue stimulation is that as noted these organs are indirectly connected to, and thus impact the clitoris. The G-spot is part of the urethral sponge and has "legs" (nerves) that attach to the clitoris, thus it too is indirectly connected to the clitoris.

The Vestibular Bulbs, a.k.a. the Clitoral Bulbs.

The vestibular bulbs are two long masses of erectile tissue located on each side of the vagina's entrance, (between the inner lips of the vagina {a.k.a. labia minora}). They're connected at the entrance of the vagina.

The vestibular bulbs *do not* include the urethral sponge and thus the U-spot. The vestibular bulbs are indirectly connected to the clitoris. They're found throughout the vestibule (the space between the two inner lips,) as well as next to the clitoris, urethra, urethral sponge, and vagina. During sexual arousal the vestibular bulbs (because they are erectile tissue) fill up with blood, causing them to become firmer. As the vestibular bulbs fill up with blood, they tighten around the vagina's entrance. This can help make the penis ejaculate sooner and send its load of semen further up into the female body. The engorged vestibular bulbs also can put pressure on parts of the clitoris. After sexual arousal subsides, the blood inside the vestibular bulb's erectile tissue is released to the circulatory system by the contractions of the orgasm. If orgasm fails to materialize, the blood usually leaves the bulbs in the ensuing hours.

Like the vestibular bulbs, (a.k.a. the clitoral bulbs,) a woman's urethral sponge is inflatable spongy tissues located in the pubic area. One side of the urethral sponge rests against the pubic bone and the other side lies against the vaginal wall.

The urethral sponge surrounds the urethra. The urethral sponge is metaphorically like a roll of soft toilet paper that surrounds its thin inner brown cardboard tube (the urethra.) The urethral sponge is located above the roof of the vagina. (If the woman is lying on her back and you're looking down at her, the roof of her vagina is the part closest to you.)

Like the vestibular bulbs, the urethral sponge is composed of erectile tissue. As part of sexual arousal it becomes swollen with blood, thus compressing the urethra. This helps prevent urination during sexual activity (along with the help of the pubococcygeus muscle.)

Inside the urethral sponge are the Skene's glands (a.k.a. paraurethral glands). Here is the source of female ejaculate. The Skene's glands surround the female urethral tube, as the male's prostate surrounds the male's urethra tube. The Skene's glands empty into the urethra and the urethra is where the female ejaculate exits the body. (The ejaculate might also back-up into her bladder.) The Skene's glands have been called the equivalent of the male prostate.

Vaginal lubrication comes from the inner walls of the vagina. It's slick and slippery. Ejaculate on the other hand originates in the Skene's glands (paraurethral glands), emerges from the urethral opening and is watery. It may be interesting to note that ejaculate consists of Prostatic Acid Phosphatase and Prostate Specific Antigen, as does male prostate fluid. Even though female ejaculate comes out via the urethra, it isn't urine. It isn't yellow, it does not smell like urine and doesn't have the same chemical composition as urine.

The vagina doesn't need female ejaculation for lubrication. The vagina mainly lubricates itself via the walls of the vagina. As female ejaculation typically occurs well after sex has begun, how important to the sex act it is, remains in question. The base fluid used in the ejaculate is pulled from the circulatory system (blood), thus there's a very large source of liquid for women's bodies to make ejaculate from.

Women may squirt sometimes, or quite a bit more often. A certain number of women can be trained to ejaculate.

In traditional Chinese medicine, female ejaculate is called White Moon Flower. In ancient India, it can be known as the Nectar of Life or sacred Amrita.

The Urethral Sponge

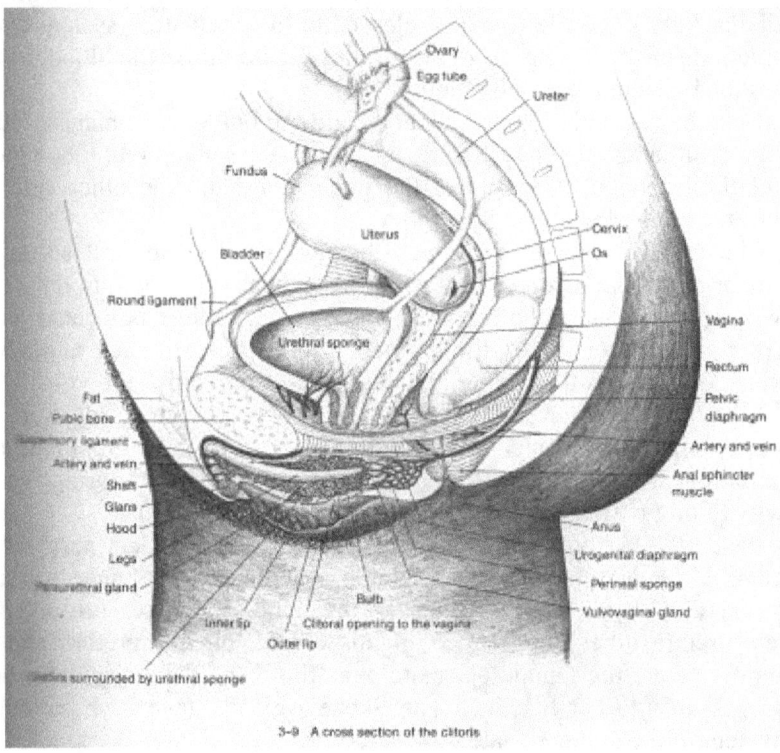

3-9   A cross section of the clitoris

The urethral sponge is made up of both erectile and glandular tissue. It has numerous nerve endings which are stimulated via the front wall of the vagina. (The front {top} wall of the vagina is what you look down at if a woman is laying on her back and you're looking down at her pubic area.) While some women derive great pleasure from stimulation of their urethral sponges, others find it irritating.

Since the urethral sponge encompasses the clitoral nerve, stimulation of the clitoris may activate the nerve endings of the urethral sponge, and vice versa. During rear-entry sex the penis is often angled slightly downward and can stimulate the front wall of the vagina more this way, (thus the urethral sponge,) Because of this some women get more U-spot related pleasure from the rear-entry position.

Under the clitoral hood (called the prepuce) and the skin of the labia, are hundreds of tiny glands that provide secretions to protect those nearby delicate areas from friction. Those areas include the exposed portion of the urethral sponge.

The G-spot

Like the U-spot, the G-spot (Gräfenberg Spot) is found in (on) the urethral sponge. The G-spot (though there is some debate as to it's existence) is located up to 3 inches (2.5–7.6 cm) up the same front (top) vaginal wall mentioned earlier. With the proper sexual stimulation it can expand into the vagina and make a "bump" that can be stimulated. The G-spot is connected to the clitoris via nerves (sometimes called "legs") and thus can also provide pleasure by tapping onto the clitoris' amazing orgasmic abilities.

Here is one of the suggested ways to find your G-spot. **Make sure you're quite sexually aroused. If you have a G-spot, this likely will make the G-spot protrude into the vagina a bit.** Insert one or two fingers (a vibrating curved tip toy may work better) two inches into the vagina and starting at the top of the vagina, exert the necessary force, or vibrating force, at the 12 o-clock position. If your G-spot doesn't make its presence known, try repeating this process further in another third of an inch, then another third of an inch and then to play it safe another third of an inch and maybe another third. If it hasn't made its presence felt yet, do the same procedure, but starting from two inches in at the 12:30 position and if necessary then again at the 1:00 position. If the G-spot remains hidden try this procedure in the 11:30 position and the 11:00 o'clock position. There are reports of women finding their G-spots in the 10:00, 10:30, 1:30 and 2:00 position. Again you want to start testing from two inches into the vagina (or maybe start at 1 inch to play it safe) and then further and further into your vagina. Most G-spots, if they're found, are found 2-3 inches in from the front of the vagina, but yours might very well be located outside those parameters. Please note that you may be one of the hundreds of millions of women who don't have a G-spot and there remains some doubt in academic circles as to whether it really even exists.

Urethral Intercourse

Urethral intercourse is not associated with the urethral sponge or the U-spot.

Urethral intercourse is the unadvised penetration of the female urethra by an object associated with sexual activity. It can result in loss of urethral sphincter control.

A Foley catheter (indwelling urinary catheter) is a catheter that can be inserted into a women's who wants to engage in very prolong sexual intercourse, often with multiple partners (such as at gangbangs.) It stays inserted through her urethra by means of a balloon at the tip, which is inflated with sterile water.

Where the U-spot is and How to Stimulate It

The U-spot (which is on the exposed portion of the urethral sponge as we found out earlier) first needs to be found on a woman and then coaxed into giving as much pleasure as possible. A significant number of women won't achieve orgasm from U-spot stimulation but will instead get a pleasant sensation. U-spot orgasms however can start occurring at anytime. **Important - when first searching for her U-spot, make sure she's already quite sexually stimulated.**

This small area of sensitive erectile tissue is often located around the urethral opening. It may however not be there but be close by that area instead. It can vary in size and be on both sides of the urethra, just above it or below it. There can even appear to be more than one U-spot. The wet tongue (or tongue tip,) lubricated tip of the penis, or lubricated finger can be used to stroke it lightly. (Gentle stroking is typically more pleasurable than pushing on it. Make sure your finger nails are well manicured.) As this erogenous zone is easier to see without special equipment, it's often easier to find the U-spot than the A-spot and G-spot.

The easiest way to find the U-spot via oral sex is to first locate the outer roof of her vagina with your tongue, then softly and slowly lick with the tongue or tongue tip upwards (outside of her vagina) towards the clitoris. If you've gotten to her clitoris without U-spot activation then you've gone too far. Remember the U-spot isn't necessarily straight up from the vagina to the urethra but could well be somewhat off to a side. Chances are it's small so use the tip of your tongue. Another way is to vibrate your tongue tip (instead of licking) in the area just discussed. The closer you get to her urethra the more likely it is to make it's appearance.

Oral sex may be the best way to find and/or stimulate the U-spot. One, the mouth provides plenty of lubrication, two, the tongue has a nice range of movement, three, the tongue has a tip to look for a potentially small sized U-spot, and four, women tend to like oral sex anyway.

Many women have discovered this spot when their lover rubbed his penis or mouth up and down their pubic area. Stimulating both the U-spot and clitoris simultaneously can provide a heightened sexual experience.

Some women have very sensitive U-spots, while some don't. It may take many attempts to find the U-spot. When using lubricated fingers, you may find she likes to have some wet stroking all the way from the clitoris, over the U-spot, and then just into the opening of the vagina. Just remember to first try lightly touching the area, not pushing on it. A small tip vibrator may work best (like a G-spot vibrator.) If you can stimulate both her U-spot and clitoris simultaneously, wow will she ever be grateful!

Once you've found her U-spot you can experiment with going faster or slower and/or using different amounts of pressure.

The End

Absolutely Essential Tips for Buying & Selling On eBay

Copyright 2014

*eBay is a registered trademark of eBay Inc.

Book #5

Important Tips for **Buying** on eBay

1) Last Minute Bidding Frenzies - Perhaps you've noticed that often there's a bidding frenzy in the last one minute of bidding. New bidders may suddenly start bidding in the hope that the previous bidders will not be watching or can't increase their bid in time. Often however it's because of *Sniping.*

Sniping websites automatically bid on your behalf, often in the last 10ish seconds. Simply sign up, enter an eBay item number and the maximum price you're willing to pay. Hidbid.com and goofbid.com offer sniping services that place bids for you.

Typically you'll need to give sniping sites your eBay password for them to work (ugh!!) Obviously that is a serious security concern.

There's little protection from eBay if things go wrong when sniping, since you willingly gave your password to a third party. If you do sign up for such a service, never use the same password for eBay as you use for other accounts like banks accounts or email addresses.

2) Second-chance Auction Scams, Beware of Them - Unscrupulous people sometimes watch bidders in high-dollar auctions and try to take unsuspecting buyer's money after an auction ends.

The scheme, known as a *Second-chance Auction Scam,* is just one of many types of Internet auction frauds reported to the *Internet Crime Complaint Center,* or *IC3.*

Second-chance scammers wait until auctions end and then offer bidders that lost, a phony second chance to purchase the item -- usually through a wire transfer service. This happens more often than people realize, beware!

3) Misspelling Search Tool - Typojoe.com, goofbid.com, bargainchecker.com, fatfingers.co.uk and baycrazy.com - There are many items listed on eBay every day that have misspelled words in the title. It's unfortunate for the seller but chances are good those listings will not come up well in eBay's search engine (because misspelling causes keyword problems) and thus not bring the seller top dollar. Their loss can be your gain!

4) Bidding Tip - Often sellers start auctions at .99 cents, (or at least under a dollar) hoping a bidding war will erupt. Many items go unspotted, staying at this super-low price (99 cents). *LastminuteAuction.com* hunts for eBay auctions due to finish within an hour but where the price still is very low.

With these items in particular, double-check delivery charges, as some sellers hope to recoup costs by charging a little extra (though eBay's now set maximum delivery charges for many categories).

5) Don't Forget About Facbook - Facbook Marketplace is a force to be reckoned with. Also sellers often are open to haggling. Just log on to your account at Facbook and search for "Marketplace". It's also worth checking to see if there's any local Facbook selling groups in your area.

6) Nigerian Type Scam for Paying. These unscrupulous people want to pay with a money order that they claim to already have handy. Often it's for more than the purchase amount. He writes to ask if the seller would be "honest enough" (or something of that nature) to send him the extra cash along with the item. (However he might just try to only buy the item with it and not ask for extra cash.) Unfortunately the money order can look okay but is counterfeit. They particularly like the *Buy It Now* feature.

7) Set Long-term Alerts For Rare Items - If you want something very specific or hard to find, set a 'favorite search' and eBay will email each time a seller lists your desired item.

Simply type a product in eBay's search bar, such as "silver dollar", and click 'save search'. Be as specific as possible for the most accurate results. When (and if) someone lists one, you're alerted with an email.

8) Don't Assume eBay's the Cheapest Place To Get Your Item - Many people assume that if it's on eBay, it's automatically the least expensive place to get it, but that often isn't the case. Perhaps you'd also like to use *shopbots* (shopping robots) that check numerous Internet retailers to find the best price. Type into a search engine "shopping comparison sites".

The same rule applies when buying used merchandise. Check used marketplaces on Amazon.com and Play.com - you may even get it for free on Freecycle or Freegle.

9) Check the eBay Going Rate For an Item - There's a quick way to check an eBay product's average price. Enter the item into the search box and click "completed listings". What will come up is a list of prices that similar auctions have already settled on. After that, sort it by "Price: lowest first". If the price is red, it means no one bought it. Green means it sold. Figure out the average price.

10) eBay has banned the selling of intangible items, and that includes curses! - Among the items that were prohibited as of August 30, 2012, are "advice; spells; curses; hexing; conjuring; magic; prayers; blessing services; magic potions; healing sessions; work from home businesses and information; wholesale lists, and drop shop lists."

11) Haggling on eBay Can Pay Off - There's nothing wrong with asking for a discount, even if the listing doesn't have the "make offer" indication. Haggling works best on *Buy It Now* listings, or auctions with a high start price and no bids. Also you'll likely do better if you haggle as the auction is coming closer to closing as the seller could start feeling more desperate.

To contact the seller, click on the seller's nickname then "ask seller a question". If you're polite, you'll likely get further. Blunt requests such as "dude, how about $15?" likely won't work out as well. Remember the seller is likely going to lose money doing this so no point in being annoying.

Once you've arranged a deal, try to keep the transaction within eBay. Ask the seller to add (or change) a Buy It Now price. That way you don't lose the usual eBay buyer protection privileges.

12) Other Things to Do To Exploit Sellers' Screw-ups - Some sellers make basic mistakes, leavings goods going for bargain money.

As well as spelling boo-boos, another error is to leave out key details such as shoe size, dress brand, saying a console's an a Wii when the photo shows a Xbox. At this point, many buyers give it up as "too much hassle".

So contact the seller to fill in gaps, but don't ask the question via the item's listing page, (because that way, when the seller replies, eBay lets them add their reply to the main listing, so it's no longer your secret.)

Instead, ask the question via the seller's profile (make it clear which item you're talking about). They might not bother with the extra hassle of adding it to the listing, so you'll be the only one in the know.

Also the seller might not realize how pricy an item he/she actually has.

13) Tool to Track Down Crazy End Times - Listings that finish at anti-social times often get fewer bids, thus sell for less. To locate auctions that finish when fewer people are around to bid on them, use BayCrazy's *Crazy End Time* search. (A lot more on the best times to end your auction in the next section of the book "*Selling on eBay*".)

Check out their auto-bidding tools if you don't want to spend all that time in front of the computer bidding at odd times. Other BayCrazy.com tools include "unwanted gift" and "ending now" searches. www.baycrazy.com/search.php?page=nightowl (Baycrazy offers other eBay related opportunities also.)

14) Search Descriptions as Well as Titles - eBay automatically searches seller's titles for results that include your specified keywords. If you're not getting the results you want, try also searching the item's *description* too. (To do this go to Advanced Search.)

For example, imagine you were searching for a REI Jacket. Unfortunately the seller may be selling one but only put "Ski Jacket" in the title however he mentioned "REI" in the description. Include description in your search and then it should then come up.

15) Search Using eBay Boolean Logic - If a seller could describe an item different ways, you can make eBay search for several different ways of describing it at once. Just place "((" at the beginning and enter different phrases individually enclosed by quotation marks, then followed by commas.

So for example, type... (("fishing tackle", "hook", "reel" ...and it will simultaneously bring up listings that contain the words "fishing tackle", "hook" and/or "reel".

16) Add A Few Extra Cents to Your Bid - When bidding, you enter a "maximum bid", and eBay makes automatic bids on your behalf up to your maximum bid.

Don't enter a round number. For example, if a coat is currently selling for $20, and the most you are willing to pay for it is $25, enter a maximum bid of $25.24. If someone tries to outbid you by entering the round number of $25, they will receive an outbid notice. eBay will go your bid, even though it's just 24 cents more.

17) Be Somewhat Skeptical of Feedback - eBay sellers have a feedback rating that acts as a useful guide to previous seller's opinion's of them. As a guideline, look for a seller with more than 98% positive feedback and a high feedback score of at least 30. Also ensure you read their feedback from their *selling*, not just their *buying*. (To see their feedback, click on their username).

18) Seller with Zero Feedback Could be Cause For Concern - Think twice before purchasing expensive items from a seller with zero feedback.

Remember feedback's useful but not infallible. One thing to watch for is traders selling a number of cheap things for $1ish each to build their feedback, and suddenly listing items costing hundreds each.

19) Check to Make Sure You're Bidding on the Actual Item - Sometimes you assume you're bidding for an item on eBay (or any auction site,) when all that's actually being sold is a link to another site selling it. People are not suppose to be able to sell these on eBay but they can fall through the cracks.

Always read the whole description in detail before bidding. Often the catch is hidden in the text at the end – an attempt to protect the seller from any recourse.

20) Scam - Beware of it - It's a red flag if a seller writes "Before bidding, contact me" then asks for a money transfer. Thieves who hijack actual eBay accounts might use this tactic.

21) Scam - Beware of it - Always be worried if you're asked to pay by an instant money transfer service such as Western Union or MoneyGram. Instant money transfer payments cannot be traced and are highly popular with thieves.

22) Sneakily Find Underpriced Buy It Nows - Feel free to hunt for Buy It Now bargains also. Perhaps the seller under-values their item making their price a good deal.

These steals are snapped up quickly. Go to "Advanced Search", select a category you're interested in, filter it to show *Buy It Now* items and sort the results.

23) Always Complain within 45 Days - Under eBay's buyer protection program, 45 days is the most number of days you have to open a case if you're unhappy with your purchase. (There are some exceptions such as tickets for events that are months away.) Read more on eBay's protection policy.
http://pages.ebay.com/help/policies/buyer-protection.html#conditions1

Under eBay's own Buyer Protection rules, buyers are eligible for a refund if the item's "not as described", meaning it didn't match the seller's description. http://pages.ebay.com/coverage/index.html

24) Pay by PayPal - Avoid sending checks and never use money orders. It's much harder for scammers to disappear with your cash when you use eBay's online payment system, PayPal.

Paying this way costs the same as paying by check, but means you're covered by eBay's Buyer Protection program. If an item is faulty, counterfeit or non-existent, you are far more likely to get a refund.

25) Outbid? Don't Give Up On It Yet - Missed out on a desired item by pennies? Don't give up hope. As every seller knows, sales sometimes don't materialize when buyers change their minds or can't come up with the dough. Because of that feel free to send a friendly message such as: "Hi, I've been looking for this poster for years and just saw your finished auction. Please let me know if the sale doesn't come through."

They may send a *Second-chance Offer*, which are sent out by sellers to unsuccessful bidders if the winner fails to pay up. Ask them to relist at an agreed *Buy It Now* price.

26) Know Your Consumer Rights - When buying from a person who makes or sells goods for resale on eBay you often have the same rights as when buying in person from a shop that does the same. This means your goods must be of satisfactory quality and as described.

With private sellers it's buyer beware. Buyers' only rights under law are that the product is fairly described and the owner has the right to sell it.
Under eBay's own Buyer Protection rules, buyers are eligible for a refund if the item is "not as described", meaning it doesn't match the seller's description.

27) Beware of All The Fakes - While eBay has a 'flag and remove' policy to help identify fakes, still plenty fall through the cracks.

If you're buying big-name brands, do your research first. Carefully check sellers' feedback and post on the forum's eBay board to get others' opinions. Be especially wary of overseas sellers or branded items that seem especially cheap.

The more *unprofessional* the photos, likely the better. Thieves often take professional photos from the brands' sites. Legitimate sellers typically take photos of items at home that might not come out as well.

28) Think Twice Before You Give A Seller Negative Feedback - Of course, negative feedback is often justified but have a heart, don't leave negative or even *neutral* feedback without first trying to work the issue out with the seller. Most sellers are good folks who will try to help particularly, as it can mean a lot to their business to stay in your good graces.

Remember eBay users can view the feedback you've left for others, and if you leave a significant amount of negative feedback, they may well decide you're too high of a risk to sell to.

29) Add An Item You're Interested in to eBay's "Watch List" - Want to keep track of an item without bidding on it? eBay lets you add items to a "Watch List", so you can relax knowing you'll get an email reminder within 36 hours of the auction ending. To watch an item, just click the *"add to watch list"* link in the upper part of the item's eBay webpage.

30) Don't Do Private Purchasing - Sellers may suggest you do a deal outside eBay for a cheaper price. If you do you'll likely have less protection if things go bad. You won't be able to leave negative feedback and you won't be protected by eBay's Buyer Protection Plan.

31) Think Safety When Picking Up An Item In Person - The usual precautions apply. If you get to their door and the seller's holding a butcher knife, now's the time to run.

32) Think International - There's bargains to be had on overseas eBay sites. To include foreign auctions in search results, click "worldwide" for location.

Still can't find what you want? Another option is buying directly from *international* eBay sites. The main ones are USA, Canada, Australia, Germany, France and Spain - there's a full list at the bottom of eBay's homepage. Make sure that the item reads *"Shipping to: worldwide"* before bidding as some international sellers only do business with their country's buyers.

Always factor in postage and if applicable, custom fees. Remember that return postage fees could be hefty.

Also what kind of credit card protections will there be? You're often still protected by eBay and PayPal's buyer protections (if you use PayPal), but it's worth investigating. Type in "buyer protection" in PayPal.

33) Don't Forget The Online Classified Ads - Again, let's not assume that because it's on eBay, that's where you'll get the best price for an item. Unfortunately that's often just not the case. Type "top classified ad sites" or something of that nature, into search engines. There's also *Freecycle* and *Freegle*. (Those two sites offer free stuff. freecycle.org and ilovefreegle.org.)

Remember, anyone can post on these classified ad sites. If someone asks you to pay by MoneyGram or Western Union, as always be concerned. It's a bad way to pay.

34) Check Other Auction Sites Also - There are other auction sites that can be found through search engines. If you're searching for something specific, it's also worth adding it to your search. *Auctionlotwatch*.com is a useful shopbot for online auctions. Search for an item and it trawls the big auction sites for you.

35) Check Cashback and Voucher Websites - Check cashback websites to see if there's money back available on your eBay purchase. Type into search engines: "cashback and voucher sites".

Cashback sites give you a cut of their proceeds by setting you up with product and/or service providers.

36) eBay has trained teachers that could be in your area. Also see eBay University. Check out:

http://pages.ebay.com/sellerinformation/howtosell/university.html

Important Tips for <u>Selling</u> on eBay

1) Join eBay Forums - Ask questions about anything, selling, buying etc. Great information is posted already and could be of use. Work together as a team. Find eBay and other auction forums by looking those up in search engines. Ebay has forums also. http://forums.ebay.com/category/Ebay-Discussion-Boards/2001

2) eBay Research Tool 1 - To help in your research about selling items, you can go Type into a search engine "best selling eBay items." EBay provides that information.

3) eBay Research Tool 2 - You can use Ebuyers (www.ebuyersedge.com) to just search eBay for items as well as set up a saved eBay search (or a number of them). You'll get alerted with an e-mail when a matching item is listed.

4) Sell Refurbished Products - Refurbished products fall somewhere in between new and used products. Refurbished products are not new, but often they aren't significantly used either. Sometimes a customer buys the product and for whatever reason, returns it for a refund. The item is then returned to the manufacturer, given an inspection, repaired as necessary and sold as refurbished.

There are various ways an item can become refurbished.

1. The packaging of an item can be damaged during shipping. In that case the item is sent back to the seller/manufacturer. Refurbished items usually come with manufacturer's warranties. Although sometimes the warranties that come with refurbished items are for a shorter period of time, the products are usually in very good condition.

2. Items that have a slight defect or flaw, like a scratch or mechanical flaw, might be returned to the manufacturer. The manufacturer repairs the items, repackages them and marks them refurbished.

3. Demonstration units are also considered refurbished, but generally that's when they're returned to the manufacturer, inspected and repackaged.

4. Brand new overstock items can also be marked refurbished.

5. Sometimes it's a situation where only the packaging of an item is opened. It's re-packaged or even just closed up and marked as refurbished.

Refurbished Products Advantages:

a. Refurbished products are significantly cheaper than new products. They also come with warranties, boxes and everything else new products come with.

b. Selling refurbished products is more profitable, even though refurbished products cost significantly less than new products. On eBay (and at other places) refurbished products can sell for the same price as new ones. (Many people buy refurbished products thinking they're buying new ones.)

c. Refurbished products are sometimes new! When you buy a lot of refurbished products they might actually be overstock items or factory overruns. In that case you would be buying new products at a fraction of the price.

Refurbished Products Disadvantages:

a. Refurbished is not new, even though refurbished products can be exactly the same as new ones, people simply prefer new items.

b. Refurbished products are sometimes the previous year's models. If you're selling electronics or computers it could bring the selling prices down.

5) Finding Products To Sell - Unfortunately finding products to sell can be the toughest part of starting your eBay business. Many people end up opting against starting an eBay business because they can't find a good supplier.

a) YELLOWPAGES.COM - www.yellowpages.com. Try this first. Yellowpages.com can find specialized suppliers in your area. Type in "wholesale" into the search box and you will be given a bunch of subdirectories to further explore. Make sure the search is based on a location near you. Next type "wholesale directory" or "wholesale directories" into search engines.

When searching also try inputting keywords such as overstock, salvage, surplus, liquidation, auction, refurbished, refurb, supplier, closeout, wholesale, etc.

b) BUY FROM AN ACTUAL EBAY SELLER. Buy multiple items and get a discount. That discount could be your margin of profit.

c) BUY WHOLESALE LOTS FROM EBAY AND RESALE THEM - Go to eBay and search for "wholesale lot". If you buy a big lot, you could find you profit best by individually selling the items in the big lot.

d) PERHAPS SELL DIGITAL COUPONS. You should be able to get them for free. As of this writing, people are posting that coupons sell well on eBay. If you're selling coupons, you need to mention that your auction is for the time you spend finding, assembling (sorting) and sending the coupons to the buyer rather than selling the coupons themselves. It's illegal to sell coupons and that's why auctions say the payment is for the time to gather and sort them. Still it can take time to find good coupons and first folks need to know where to look.

e) BUY FROM LIQUIDATION COMPANIES - A liquidator is someone that buys overruns from big retailers (Sears, K-mart, Wal-Mart etc.) at a fraction of the wholesale price. Sometimes big stores can't sell everything they have. The stuff they couldn't sell needs to be gotten rid of as soon as possible to make room for new products. This is where liquidation companies come in. They buy the overruns products, often at a fraction of the wholesale price. When a liquidation company buys a couple of truckloads full of overruns, the next thing it must do is sell these overruns ASAP to make room for more overruns. Since the liquidator must get rid of the products as soon as possible, the products are sold at cheap prices and often in bulk. Perhaps there are liquidator stores in your town what would make you a deal and you wouldn't necessarily have to buy in bulk.

f) BOOK SALES - With books, you can sell a digital product that can simply be emailed to your customer. No packing and shipping involved! Selling books on eBay is easy. In fact there are systems you can implement to essentially automate the entire process. You could do a *Buy It Now* auction, or just start the bidding at a reasonable price. When the auction ends and the buyer pays you, all you need to do is email the book to them. Again, that's the great thing about downloadable information products: no packaging or shipping is necessary. Perhaps you'd like to offer an entire collection of books to sell on eBay. You'll need books that you own or have given you resale rights.

g) You can sell peoples' houses, cars, boats, or even jewelry collections. Just look in the for sale listings of your local newspaper and look at all of the great stuff for sale that would sell on eBay. Call up the owners of the items advertised in the newspaper and offer to sell the stuff for them. Looking for stuff in newspapers is great because the people that are using a newspaper to sell something probably know little about eBay and are desperate to get rid of the stuff they're advertising. These people are also the ones that are willing to lower the price and haggle, and that is great because the lower the price they are willing to let the item go for, the more profit you can make by selling their stuff.

h) RUNNING ADS TO FIND MERCHANDISE - You can run ads in print media and/or post what you're looking for in Internet forums with something like "I will buy your stuff". As previously noted, if you are going to use this method you will need to pick a used product that keeps its value well. If you're going to use this method you should buy things like jewelry and watches, antiques and other things that appreciate with age.

A previous seller's success story was selling old collectable Apple computers. This is a type of item that some people have laying around in the basement or attic, and will likely never use again. They're more than happy to unload it and get a little money for it at the same time. But on eBay it was a whole new ballgame. There are thousands of people who collect old collectable computers.

6) *Sell To Resellers* - Anyone looking to buy products and resell them to make a profit is a very good customer that will come back and buy from you again and again. Plenty of people buy stuff on eBay then resell it on eBay! There are also those who buy products on eBay to resell them on their other ecommerce websites or actual stores they may own. A lot of PowerSellers (special higher volume eBay sellers with a closer relationship to eBay) started by buying stuff off of eBay and simply putting it back up for auction.

7) *Order Samples If Possible* - This is a particularly good tip if you don't have a chance to inspect and see the products you are ordering in person. Many people starting out on eBay make the mistake of placing a big order before actually seeing what they're ordering. By ordering samples you'll be able to test not only the quality of the products you're ordering but the service, communication and legitimacy of the company you're ordering from. If you're thinking of selling designer clothing on eBay, be extra careful when ordering your supplies from the Internet. There is a lot of fake (counterfeit) clothing being sold on the Internet. Remember the pictures on the supplier's website may look real, but that doesn't mean they will be sending you what's in the picture.

If you find a great deal but the "supplier" won't allow any sample orders and wants you to pay through an untraceable method, be wary.

8) Second-chance Offers - If the buyer of your item falls through, you can send the other bidders a *Second-chance Offer* to see if they're still interested in buying it.

9) The Listing's Title - The title of your listing should be clear, relevant to what you are selling and attention grabbing. Always include the correct spelling of the item in the title. Don't try to make the title "cool" by deliberately misspelling words, unless perhaps if the slang name for it is popular. If you misspell the title, your listing won't show up in search results because presumably most people aren't searching for the slang name (or misspelled version) of the product.

The title has to be short (eBay rules), so make sure you include the name of the item and abbreviated descriptions, and try not to waste any space on words that are not needed. *By the same token, always use the entire allotted space to write your title. In general, the longer the title, the better, as long as all your keywords are relevant.*

10) Keywords & Relevancy - Make sure the brand name of what you're selling is in the title! If you're selling a Champion Portable Generator, your listing title should include the make and model number, in this case "New Champion 42431 Portable Generator, 1500 Watt". Your listing title should be a short, abbreviated description of the item you are selling.

The name of the product in the title has to do with the search results (keywords). If people want to buy your portable generator they may search "portable generator, generator, Champion, Champion portable generator," etc. You want to make your listing show up in as many search results as possible.

In review, a wild but catchy title will definitely grab the attention of most people who see it, but won't come up in many people's search results, unless also in the title listing is the name of the product that people would type in when looking for it. (Even that's not guaranteed to work.)

11) If a potential customer wants other people's opinions on a product you sell, you might want to send them to the Amazon.com's webpage for the site as Amazon posts feedback from buyers of that same product. Make sure that Amazon is not selling it for less than you are or that idea could backfire!

12) Mention Flaws: If there is a flaw in the item you are selling, make sure you mention it (though try to call it something else like "scratch" or "mark" if that's what it is.) If your product has a flaw and you don't mention it in your listing, you could get negative feedback and a request for a refund from the person who buys the "flawed" item.

If possible, make the flaw sound positive. You could say "this product has a small dent that has no effects on its operation, but because of this you save big bucks!"

Mentioning a flaw also can make you look like an honest person. You can even have the flaw mentioned in your bullet points - Small scratch on the top (saves you money!!)

13) Host Your Own Pictures - You can host your own pictures on another website or your eBay Store and thus show many, many more photos free of charge.

14) Payment Options: - You should offer the customer several different choices of payment. Most of your customers will pay you through PayPal so make sure you get a PayPal account (www.PayPal.com). Some may prefer Western union's Bidpay. Another one is *Skrill.com.*

Paypal does not service a lot of foreign countries. Call them to find out which ones they're not currently servicing.

Wire Transfers - Unscrupulous overseas buyers prefer these as they're not as traceable. It's preferable not to take them.

15) Offering SquareTrade Warranties - If applicable to what you're selling, another good way to build trust is to sign up for SquareTrade warranties at www.squaretrade.com. www.squaretrade.com/seller-faq

16) About Me Page - The About Me page is often overlooked by many eBay sellers (and buyers.) While having the free About Me page likely will not dramatically increase your sales, it can help if you have good things to say about yourself and a nice picture. Note, many sellers only include links to their listings and maybe not enough information about themselves in the About Me page.

17) People Bidding with 0 Feedback ratings - Having a good to great feedback rating is so important as you know. Many sellers refuse letting members with 0 feedback bid on their auctions. Getting a negative feedback from somebody that unpredictable is simply a risk we don't want to take. In many cases, we simply don't trust them.

18) Best Time To End Your Auction - The best time for an auction to close (end) is in the evenings and on weekends as that's when most people are on the Internet for that type of activity! You want to make sure that when your auction is closing (ending), everyone that's interested in it is available to bid on it. The mornings are the times that the eBay website gets the least visitors (as people are more often sleeping or working.)

If you live in the Eastern Time Zone, list your auction between 9pm-11pm, Central Time Zone list between 8-10pm, Mountain Time Zone between 7-9pm, and for the Pacific Time Zone list between 6-8pm. This will give you the biggest exposure at the end of your auction. The debate is out as to what day your auction should end on. Some sellers report that Tuesday, Wednesday and Thursday are best. Other sellers report that Saturday and Sunday are best.

There are a few exceptions though. For example, some business products sell best during weekdays and during work hours. Obviously this is because people are usually ordering those types of products at work, for work. Studies have shown that a listing that ends at peak hours can attract up to 25% more bids than one that ends in non-peak hours. Listing your auctions at optimal times is one of the easiest ways to attract more bids.
To end the auction in the evenings, you'll need to put the item for sale in the evening (*or use listing software [see next page] to do it for you*) as eBay considers each day to have a length of 24 hours.

Note, it's eBay's practice that when someone's auction is ending, that listing shows up higher on keyword search results (which is a good thing!)

19) Terms of Service Webpage (Yours) - That's something even a lot of experienced sellers don't seem to include, though it likely won't be necessary if all the information is already in your FAQ webpage. For instance, what's the return policy? What are the shipping options, and what will they cost? What are the accepted methods of payment? How soon is payment to be sent? What is the warranty?

20) Listing Software (For Your Items) - Listing software organizes your eBay listings making the listing part of your business simpler and more efficient. There are many different kinds of listing software. You can do an Internet search for them.

Turbo Lister is free software from eBay. Turbo Lister allows you to upload thousands of listings at a time. It saves listings, schedules your listings and uploads them to eBay automatically. Using it you can edit multiple listings at the same time, preview what your listings will look like before uploading them and more. More eBay software is offered at:

http://pages.ebay.com/help/sell/advanced_selling_tools.html

21) Drop Shipping What You Sell - With drop shipping all you have to do is list items up for auction and when they sell, you contact your supplier, who ships the products from their factory, straight to your customers. In theory drop shipping is a good way to go, but it could offer problems. What happens when you sell items and your supplier sends them to the wrong addresses? What happens when you sell items and your supplier is out of stock? In those cases your reputation suffers. If you are going to use drop shipping; make sure there is good communication between you and your supplier (drop shipper.) Also make sure you have some products in stock in case the supplier runs out by the time your auctions have closed.

22) eBay Stores - eBay stores can be great if you have a number of items to sell. First you'll need to reach the minimum number of feedbacks required (10) to open one. Most PowerSellers have eBay stores. Store sellers can see an increase in profit of up to 25% in the first three months of opening the store (according to eBay). Having your own eBay store can save you a substantial amount of money in listing fees and let you sell items in a fixed price format as well as selling via auctions. Also you can list items for a much longer time and store them in your inventory list for 30, 60, 90, 120 days and even "Good till Cancelled". You can feature links to other auctions in all your listings by utilizing a cross promotion tool. There are also bonuses like your own search engine and monthly reports from eBay featuring statistics and dada about your sales in the past month.

An eBay store also gives you a location. It gives you a base of operation, a place where people can easily find you, and a place where repeat customers can come back to. Your customers will be able to bookmark and return to your store, and it may also be indexed in the major search engines. So if you're selling silver dollars, and someone does a BING search for silver dollars, your eBay store may appear in the results along with the usual online retail websites! Obviously this can increase your traffic greatly, and likewise boost your sales.

23) Your eBay Store Identity - Ideally your eBay store should look different from your competition. You can use the design templates eBay offer you, but perhaps it's best to use original graphics. Fortunately eBay Stores are customizable. Ideally, to establish your name, your eBay store should appear like your listings as much as possible. Same colors, design and look.

24) Get a Domain Name - You need to get a simple and memorable domain name. A domain name makes it simple for people to find you. The standard web address eBay will give to your store will look like this: *stores.ebay.com/yourname*, this is not a very memorable web address and it's too long to be easy to type into a web browser. It would be best if you had a web address like *mystore.com*.

The End

www.ingramcontent.com/pod-product-compliance
Lightning Source LLC
Chambersburg PA
CBHW070229290526
45789CB00004B/1546